5 minute first aid

life-saving skills

British Red Cross
Caring for people in crisis

5 minute first aid

life-saving skills

Hodder Arnold
A MEMBER OF THE HODDER HEADLINE GROUP

Orders: Please contact Bookpoint Ltd, 130 Milton Park, Abingdon, Oxon OX14 4SB. Telephone: (44) 01235 827720, Fax: (44) 01235 400454. Lines are open from 9.00 to 18.00, Monday to Saturday, with a 24-hour message answering service. You can also order through our website www.hoddereducation.com

British Library Cataloguing in Publication Data
A catalogue record for this title is available from the British Library.

ISBN-10: 0 340 90462 3
ISBN-13: 9 780340 904626

First published 2005
Impression number 10 9 8 7 6 5 4 3 2 1
Year 2008 2007 2006 2005

Typeset by Transet Limited, Coventry, England.
Printed in Great Britain for Hodder Arnold, a division of Hodder Headline, 338 Euston Road, London NW1 3BH, by Cox & Wyman Ltd, Reading, Berkshire.

Hodder Headline's policy is to use papers that are natural, renewable and recyclable products and made from wood grown in sustainable forests. The logging and manufacturing processes are expected to conform to the environmental regulations of the country of origin.

contents

acknowledgements **vii**
preface **ix**
introduction **xiii**

1 how to approach an emergency situation **1**
common scenarios 2
managing the situation 6
calling the emergency services 7
anxiety 8

2 what to do if a person is unconscious **12**
how to check responsiveness 13
how to open the airway 14
how to check breathing 16
how to place a person in the recovery position 18
rescue breathing 21
check for signs of circulation 23
how to do chest compressions 24

3 choking **32**
how to treat choking 32

4 severe bleeding **39**
bleeding 39
shock 43
treating shock 44
dangers of infection 46

5	**common emergency situations**	**50**
	fire	51
	road traffic accident	54
	electrical injuries in the home	56
	drowning	57
	heart attack	58
case studies		**63**
first-aid kit contents		**71**
household first-aid equipment		**75**
about the Red Cross		**79**
taking it further		**83**
index		**87**

acknowledgements

The authors would like to pay special thanks to Charlotte Hall, Catherine Jones, Genevieve Okech, Naomi Safir and Ken Sharpe.

preface

The British Red Cross, as part of the International Red Cross and Red Crescent Movement, is the world's largest first-aid training organization. With over 180 Red Cross societies worldwide we endeavour to make first-aid knowledge and skills accessible to individuals, families, schools and the wider community.

You never know when someone may need your help but it is highly likely that when called on to provide emergency first aid it will be to someone close to you such as a friend or a member of your own family. Therefore, we have produced the *Five-minute First Aid* series in order to give you the relevant skills and confidence needed to be able to save a life and help an injured person, whatever your situation.

We appreciate that it is difficult to find time in hectic lifestyles to learn first-aid skills. Consequently, this series is designed so that you can learn and absorb each specific, essential skill that is relevant to you in just five minutes, and you can pick up and put down the book as you wish. The features throughout the book will help you to reinforce what you have learnt and will build your confidence in applying first aid.

This book is divided into five-minute sections, so that you can discover each invaluable skill in just a short amount of time.

one-minute wonder

One-minute wonders ask and answer the questions that you might be thinking as you read.

key skills

The key-skill features emphasize and reiterate the main skills of the section – helping you to commit them to memory and recall them when called upon to do so.

summary

Summary sections summarize the key points of the chapter in order to further consolidate your knowledge and understanding.

self-testers

The self-testers ensure that you have learnt the most important facts of the chapter. They will give you an indication of how much you are absorbing as you go along and will help to build your confidence. (Note: some of the multiple choice questions may have more than one possible answer!)

We hope that this book will give you the opportunity to learn the most important skills you will ever need in a friendly, straightforward way and that it prepares you for any first-aid situation that you may encounter.

introduction

In recent years we, the British Red Cross, have gained a greater appreciation of the importance of providing immediate first aid for someone who has been injured or is suddenly taken ill.

You, as the first person on the scene, can carry out some important, easy-to-learn actions which will, in the most serious situation save a person's life, or in a less serious situation help the person to recover.

These prompt actions will also ensure that the injured person's condition does not deteriorate before the arrival of the emergency services. Throughout this book we will reinforce the importance of making that 999 call (or 112 in Europe) at the right time.

You never know when you may be called upon to use these first-aid skills to give first aid in an emergency situation but we in the British Red Cross know that it is highly likely that you will need to look after a friend, family member, or colleague in the workplace rather than a stranger.

Five-minute First Aid Life-Saving Skills will give you the relevant skills, knowledge and confidence to take the all-important initial steps when providing first aid in an emergency situation.

We, as authors of this book, know that it can be difficult to step out from a crowd and announce that you have some first-aid skills that will be helpful in an emergency situation. It is easy to assume that there will be someone else who will know more than you do but in our experience this is not always correct.

Therefore, this book aims to provide you with easy-to-understand guidelines that will give you the confidence to step forward and to give as much help as you can in any given emergency. To aid your understanding, we will focus on the key life-saving skills and identify the challenges that may face you in a real-life situation.

We have used this book to highlight the most common situations you are likely to encounter and present the information in a way that will help you identify the priorities and take the appropriate action.

It is important to remember that the protocols and procedures used in Chapter 2 in this book apply to older children (eight years and above) and adults. Procedures for babies and young children differ slightly and you may wish to refer to two other titles in this series: *Five-minute First Aid for Babies* and *Five-minute First Aid for Children*.

For convenience and clarity, we use the pronoun 'he' when referring to the first aider and injured person.

1

how to approach an emergency situation

We will provide you with an easy-to-understand approach to assessing any emergency situation. We will also consider occasions where there may be more than one person injured. It is important to remind you that this step-by-step approach can be used in any emergency situation including car crashes, instances of drowning, fires and electrocution.

We will also look at various scenarios you may encounter in the home, including a relative who has collapsed for no apparent reason and to whom you may need to give life-saving skills, a work colleague with a known heart condition who suddenly collapses, and a case of electrocution.

common scenarios

Let us consider a possible situation. You are at home and your elderly mother is visiting for the weekend. There has been some family discussion about her decline in health, but she does not have any known illness. She is in the sitting room watching TV and you are in the kitchen cooking dinner. You call her to come and eat but there is no response. You assume she is asleep so you call her again but she still does not reply. You go into the sitting room and find that you're unable to rouse her. She is not moving and does not respond to shouting or gentle shaking. What would you do? It is important in this situation that even if you are frightened, you must remain calm and think clearly about what to do next.

Another situation might be that you are at work, your colleague has had a period of time off sick and has confided in you that he has coronary artery disease and was off sick because he'd suffered a heart attack. On his return to work he looks well and appears to have gained his enthusiasm for work and re-established himself as part of the team. In the afternoon you notice he is not at his desk and no one in the team appears to know his whereabouts. You go to look for him and after a while you find him in the toilet lying on the floor looking pale and sweaty. What would you do?

The purpose of presenting these two scenarios is to get you thinking about how you should begin to assess the person(s) involved in an emergency situation and identify the best care. In first-aid terms this is referred to as DR ABC:

- **D** is for danger. Look for anything that may harm you, or any bystanders. Dangers may include: presence of gas, fumes, smoke, fire, electric cables, water in the case of drowning, or traffic in the case of a car crash. In any situation you, as the first aider, should never take any unacceptable risks because if you do and you injure yourself, then you will not be able to help anybody else. If there is an obvious danger and you are not able to deal with it then your first action is to call the emergency services and wait for their arrival before dealing with the incident. We cannot stress enough the importance of keeping yourself safe – first and foremost.
- **R** is for response. The term 'response' is used in first aid to describe your attempt to decide whether or not the person you are helping is awake and conscious or is not conscious. You may find that this person can make conversation and answer all your questions, however, you may find that he is drowsy, or not replying at all. If unable to respond to actions or questions, this person is clearly unconscious. If you know the person, call him by name and identify yourself to try to get some response. It is very important to know whether the person is conscious or not as this will determine what you do next.

As you will discover later in the book, you can also gently shake the person's shoulders to help you decide whether or not the person is unconscious (see Chapter 2, page 13).

- **A** is for airway. One of the most crucial parts of your assessment must be to decide whether a person has an open and clear airway. This is so important because the airway is the connecting tube between the mouth and lungs in the body. It is essential that the airway remains open in order to allow air into the lungs and provide oxygen to the body to keep the person alive. Without oxygen, the person will die and it is well known that the brain can start to become damaged after just a few minutes without oxygen. If it appears that the airway is not clear, you will need to try to remedy this before doing anything (see Chapter 2, page 14).

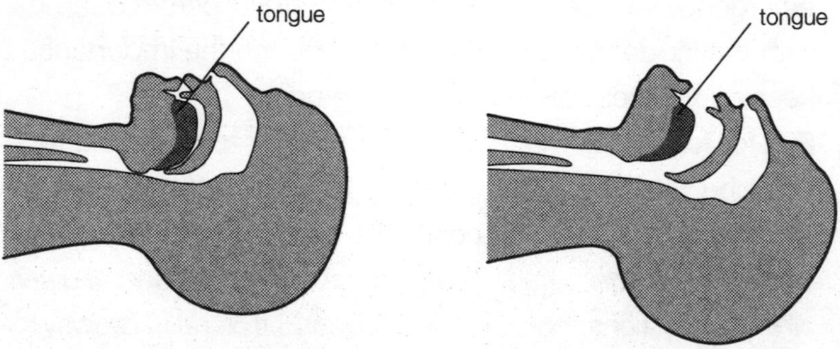

(a) Blocked airway – head not tilted (b) Unblocked airway – head tilted

Fig 1 Importance of an open airway

- **B** is for breathing. 'Breathing' is the term used to describe the movement of air in and out of the body so that the oxygen can be transferred into the bloodstream and carried around the body to keep the key organs, including the brain, heart and kidneys, alive. If the person is not breathing, this will result in a lack of oxygen in the body and you will need to breathe for the person. The air that you breathe out has some oxygen in it, which will be invaluable to a person who is not breathing (see Chapter 2, page 21 for rescue breathing).
- **C** is for circulation. This describes the continuous movement of blood around the body. The circulation flows through a series of pipes not dissimilar to the heating system in your house with the heart acting as the pump. If this circulation has stopped then you will need to simulate the work of the heart by pressing on the chest. This will result in some circulation of the blood that will carry oxygen to the key organs (see Chapter 2, page 23 for signs of circulation).

key skills

The assessment of any injured person should be based on:

- **D** danger
- **R** response
- **A** airway
- **B** breathing
- **C** circulation.

one-minute wonder

Q To avoid putting myself in danger when dealing with a car crash, is it best if I quickly move the person to the side of the road before doing my assessment?

A No. We advise that this is not good practice because the person may have life-threatening injuries. Do not move the injured person until you have carried out the assessment. Instead ask the bystanders to stop the traffic.

managing the situation

You will feel reassured if you have someone at the scene with you even if they don't know any first aid. You may also be faced with doing several tasks at once, so an extra pair of hands may be helpful. These tasks might include securing safety at the scene, calling for the emergency services or helping with first aid, especially if there is more than one person needing help. All bystanders can be helpful if given clear instructions and if they are kept busy, this will reduce the panic and confusion. If you are the most experienced first aider at the scene, you must take control and demonstrate leadership. Act with authority by giving helpers clear instructions and keeping a clear picture in mind of what is happening so that you can give clear, concise and accurate information to the emergency services when they arrive.

***one-minute** wonder*

Q What should I do if I find somebody collapsed in the street?

A Stop and help. Identify if there is someone nearby who can help you. Assess the person using DRABC and take charge of the situation until the emergency services arrive.

5 • 5

calling the emergency services

It is not possible to be definitive about when to call the emergency services, as each emergency situation is unique. However, in this book we will give you some guidelines about when to do it.

You should be aware that by dialling 999, or 112, which is the European emergency number, you will be able to access the fire service, police, ambulance, mountain rescue, fell rescue, cave rescue, mine rescue and coastguard. When you dial 999 or 112, you will be asked which service you need. If you require more than one service, please tell them, otherwise you will need to make another call.

When you make a call, the operator will ask you for information about the emergency, so it's important that you gather together certain basic information before you make the call such as your exact whereabouts and your telephone number. You will also be asked to give an indication of the seriousness of the emergency, the number of people involved and whether or not there are particular dangers such as chemical and toxic fumes.

one-minute wonder

Q If the injured person recovers after I have called the ambulance, should I cancel it?

A No, their condition may deteriorate again and it is always wise to gain a professional opinion.

anxiety

We recognize that a life-threatening emergency is a distressing experience for everyone involved. While you are dealing with the emergency you are likely to be focused on what you are doing. Once it is over and the emergency services have taken the person to hospital it is normal to reflect on what has happened and how you reacted. We know, having spoken to people in similar situations, that they have asked themselves questions like, did I do the right thing? did I call for help early enough? and what is going to happen to the person I have looked after? You may also feel upset if the emergency has resulted in a fatality. Be reassured that all of these reactions and feelings are understandable and quite normal.

In order to face up to these mixed emotions, you should talk about your feelings with friends, family or colleagues. Be aware, however, that the confidentiality of the ill person is important, so you should not talk to others about the person involved by using their name or other personal identification.

Whilst first aid is often portrayed as a heroic act, it is important that everyone realizes that the outcome of any life-threatening emergency can be either good or bad. You must realize that your willingness to act and become involved is crucial, whatever the final outcome.

summary

If you are the first person on the scene of any emergency situation:

- don't walk by
- get involved
- try and remain calm
- remember the DR ABC procedure when carrying out an assessment
- take charge and ask bystanders to help
- dial 999 (or 112 in Europe)
- do not take unacceptable risks.

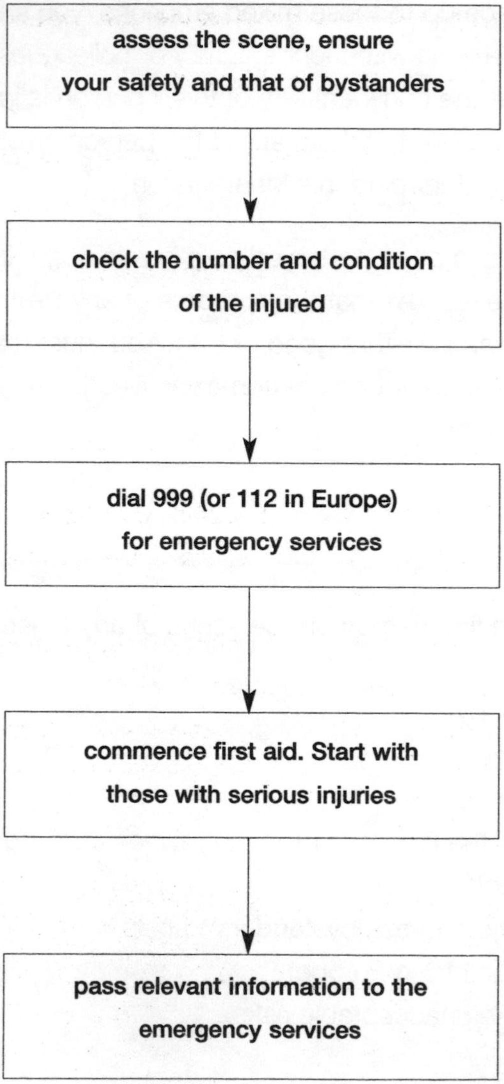

On approaching an emergency situation

self-testers

1 What do the initials DR ABC stand for?

2 Give three possible dangers you may want to consider in an emergency situation.

3 In your own words, describe your understanding of the term 'airway' as used in this chapter.

4 What is the function of circulation?

answers

1 **D**anger; **R**esponse; **A**irway; **B**reathing; **C**irculation
2 any of the following: gas; fumes; fire; smoke; electric cables; water with strong currents; traffic
3 the term 'airway' is used to describe the tube that carries air from the mouth and nose to the lungs
4 to carry blood around the body in a network of pipes

2

what to do if a person is unconscious

There are many causes of unconsciousness including stroke, head injury and diabetes. Our aim in this chapter is to highlight what you should do to help an unconscious person rather than focusing on the cause of the unconsciousness. When you come across an unconscious person it is not important in the first instance to spend time trying to find out why the person is unconscious. Instead, you should carry out the DR ABC assessment of the person (see Chapter 1) so that, if necessary, you can use your life-saving skills. It is only once you have done this that you may have the opportunity to find out what has happened. In the vast majority of situations, the cause of the unconsciousness does not impact on how you respond as a first aider. The reasons why a person is unconscious can be complex, therefore, your efforts must be focused on the assessment and management of the unconscious person.

In this chapter we will focus on the key skills needed to manage a first-aid situation and how to improve the individual's recovery.

how to check responsiveness

As you approach the person, call his name if you know it or ask 'are you alright?' Speak clearly and directly to the person, and then gently shake the person's shoulders. You may already have a picture in your mind of an unconscious person lying on the ground, but it is worth remembering that an unconscious person could also be sitting or slouched in a chair.

If there is no response, you should assume that the person is unconscious. Call out for someone to come and help you. Be prepared to shout as loud as possible to attract attention, because even if you think you are alone with the person, it is possible that there may be someone not far away who may be able to help you. It is important to get someone else to help if at all possible as they will be able to do things while you look after the injured person, such as direct traffic or phone the emergency services.

If the injured person does not respond, check that the airway is open.

how to open the airway

When a person becomes unconscious, the muscles relax and the body becomes floppy. The tendency is for the head to fall forwards and the tongue (which is also a muscle) to fall back into the throat and potentially block off the airway. This is particularly true if the person ends up lying on his back. If the tongue falls back into the throat and blocks the airway, the person cannot breath. As breathing is essential to sustain life, anything that interferes with this, like the tongue in the throat, needs to be dealt with very quickly.

key skills

How to open the airway:

- first, place one hand on the forehead to steady the head and gently tilt the head backwards. At this stage, the mouth will fall open if a person is unconscious.
- if there is any obvious obstruction in or around the mouth such as displaced dentures or a gum shield, remove it.
- using the fingertips of your other hand under the casualty's chin, lift the chin to complete the head tilt–chin tilt manoeuvre. This action brings the tongue back into its normal position in the floor of the mouth and the airway opens.

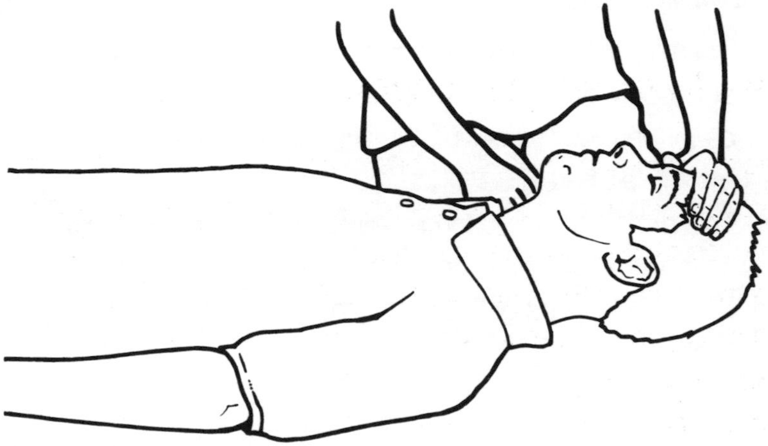

Fig 2 Opening the airway
Place one hand on the person's forehead and gently tilt the head back.

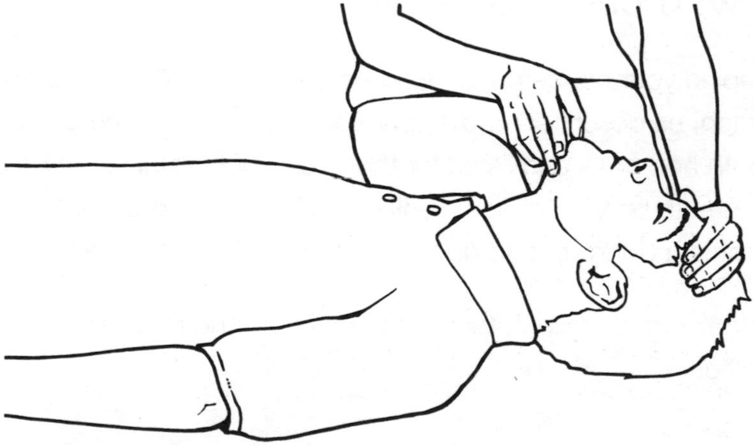

Fig 3 Lift the chin using your fingertips so that the airway opens

one-minute wonder

Q I was taught in a first-aid course, in 1986, that you should put your finger in the mouth to feel for anything that may be in the mouth blocking the airway. Why is this not mentioned here?

A This procedure is no longer advised. The 'finger sweep', as it was known, resulted in a delay in opening the airway, and the chances of finding anything in the mouth were very small.

how to check breathing

Keeping your hands on the forehead and under the chin of the person, as described above, put your ear over the person's mouth and nose and listen for the sound of breathing. Feel for the breath on your cheek. Look along the body to see if the chest is moving up and down. Do this for about ten seconds.

If breathing is present, turn the person into the recovery position.

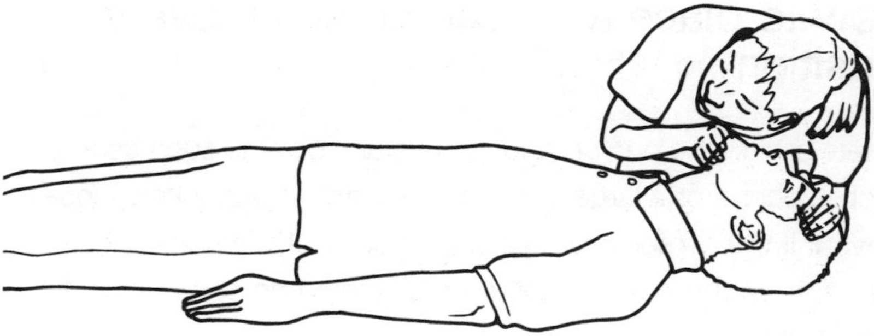

Fig 4 Check for signs of breathing

key skills

To check if a person is breathing, place your head close to the person's mouth and nose. Look, listen and feel for breathing. Do not rush this procedure.

how to place a person in the recovery position

Kneel beside the person and remove any objects such as a mobile phone or a large bunch of keys from the pockets closest to you. If the person is wearing spectacles, it's important that you remove these so as not to break them and cause injury to the person.

Take the arm that is nearest to you, bend it at the shoulder and elbow, placing the palm upwards at a right angle to the body. Then bring the other arm across the person's body, take hold of the hand and place it palm outwards against the person's cheek closest to you. If the person is wearing large rings, rotate them so that the bulky part of the ring is in the palm. Keep holding the hand against the cheek and, with your other hand, take hold of the leg furthest away from you just above the knee and pull it up until the foot is flat on the floor. Then if you pull on the knee, the person will roll towards you. You may need to move back slightly so that you can adjust the upper leg into a position with the knee bent. This action will put the person into a stable position and he will not roll any further towards you. The final adjustment should be to make sure that the person's head is tilted back and the airway is open. (See Figures 5, 6, 7 and 8.) This is the safest position for an unconscious person because if the person is sick, the vomit will drain away, as will blood, and the airway will stay open.

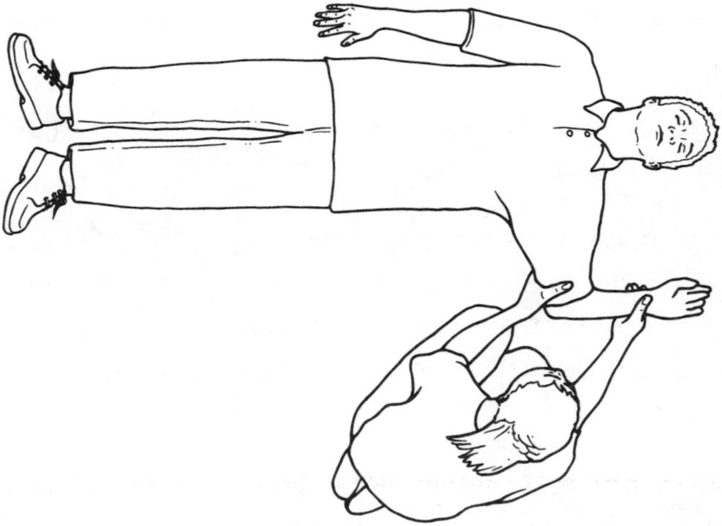

Fig 5 The recovery position
Take the person's arm closest to you, bend it at the shoulder and elbow, placing the palm upwards at a right angle to the body.

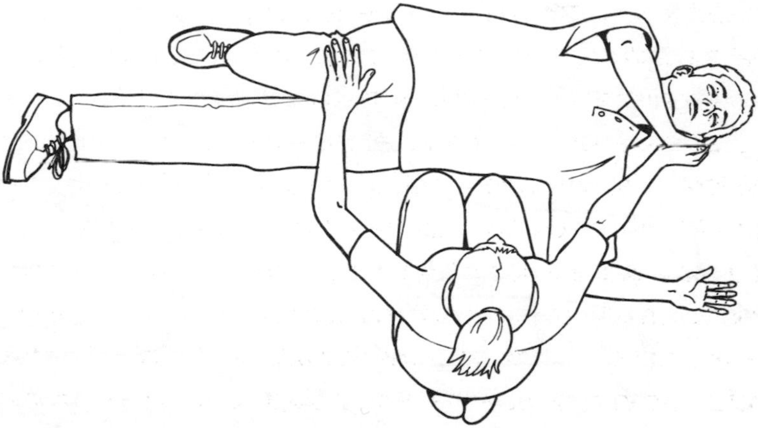

Fig 6 Take the person's furthest hand and place it palm outwards against his nearest cheek. Take the person's furthest knee and bend it until the foot is flat on the floor.

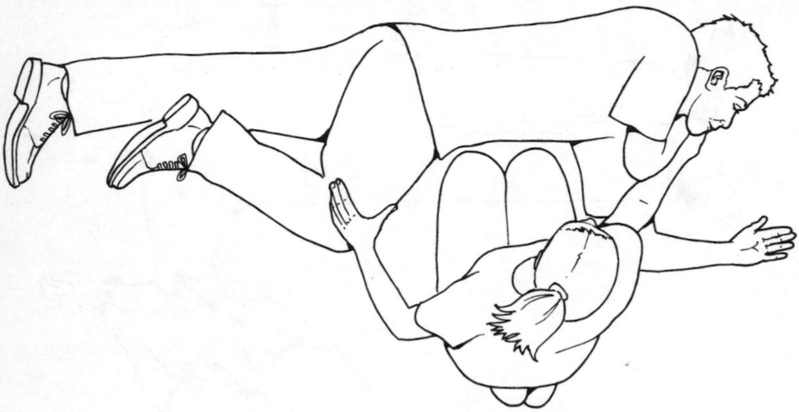

Fig 7 Using the knee as a lever, gently pull the person over towards you while continuing to support the head.

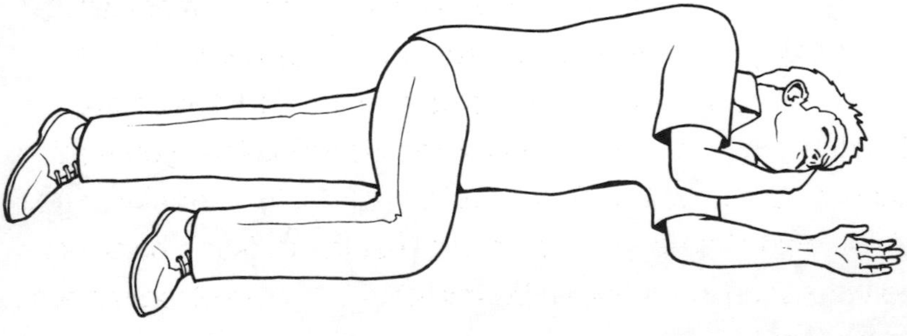

Fig 8 Once the person is securely on his side, adjust the chin and head to ensure an open airway and reposition the upper leg as shown. This is the recovery position.

key skills

For an unconscious person who is breathing, place in the recovery position and call for an ambulance.

one-minute wonder

Q If I am on my own and need to go to the telephone to call the emergency services, is it safe to leave the person in the recovery position?

A Yes. By putting the person into the recovery position, you have made him as safe as you possibly can.

rescue breathing

If the person is not breathing, you must call for an ambulance immediately. Once you have made the phone call to the emergency services you must start breathing for the person. This technique is now known as 'rescue breathing', you may know it as 'the kiss of life' or 'mouth-to-mouth ventilation'. Your aim in doing this is to try to ensure that the person's body has some oxygen in it that can be transferred via the blood stream to the key organs.

You must initially give two rescue breaths. You may feel so nervous about giving these two rescue breaths that your first rescue breath isn't successful. You are allowed five attempts to give these two initial rescue breaths. The key movement that you should look for in the person is that when you blow into the mouth, the chest rises and when you take the mouth away, the chest falls.

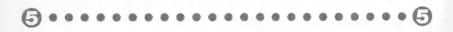

how to give rescue breaths

Kneel alongside the person and ensure the airway is open. Bring your hand down from their forehead and pinch their nose tightly. Take a breath and then place your mouth around the person's mouth and blow steadily and gently. Take your mouth away and watch the chest fall. There is no need to rush this procedure. Allow the chest to rise and fall.

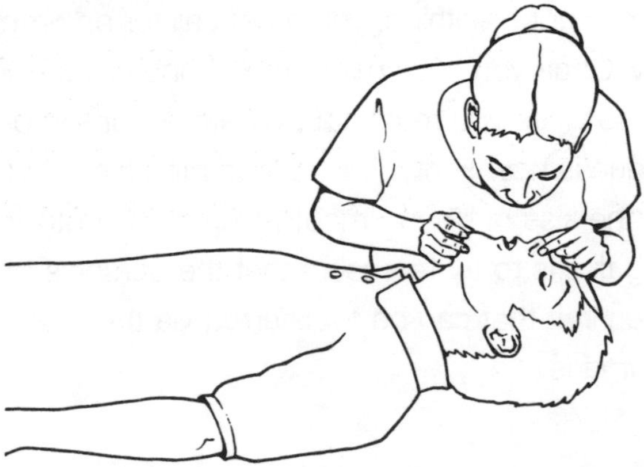

Fig 9 Giving rescue breaths
Open the airway, pinch the nose and blow gently into the person's mouth

one-minute wonder

Q Is there a risk of infection when doing rescue breathing?

A Most first-aid procedures contain an element of risk but this is very small in the case of rescue breathing. However, if you want to reduce the risk of infection, and if it is available a face shield can be used. (See first-aid kit, page 73.)

key skills

To give rescue breaths, tilt the person's head back, pinch the nose, place your mouth over his mouth and blow.

5 5

check for signs of circulation

After the initial rescue breaths, do a quick check for signs of circulation. Signs to look for include breathing, coughing or movement of the body or limbs. If there are none of these signs present then you should start chest compressions (see overleaf).

one-minute wonder

Q When I was on a course, I was advised that you should check the person's pulse to see if there is any sign of circulation. You do not mention this here. Should I do it?

A In an emergency situation it is extremely difficult to detect a pulse in a collapsed person. Even health-care professionals find it difficult. Therefore, in the context of first aid, we recommend that you check for the more obvious signs of circulation as described above, such as breathing or coughing, and don't waste time trying to find a pulse.

how to do chest compressions

This is the term used for pressing on a person's chest or doing chest pumps to simulate the work of the heart.

To carry out chest compressions kneel alongside the person and find the inverted V-notch at the bottom of the breastbone.

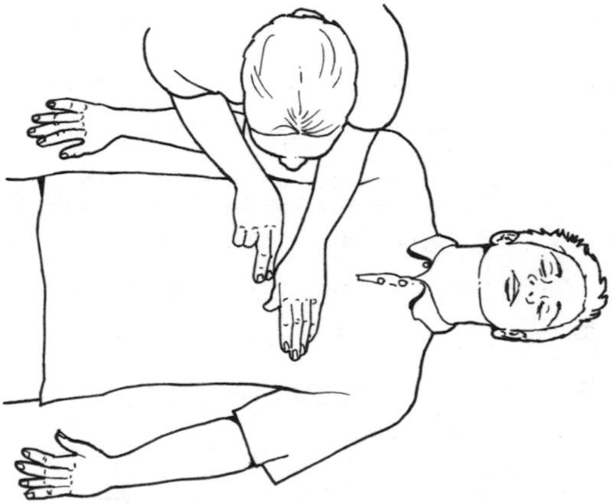

Fig 10 Performing chest compressions
Place two fingers at the end of the breastbone above the V-notch. Place the heel of your other hand alongside.

Place two fingers on the breastbone just above the notch and place the heel of the other hand on the breastbone alongside these two fingers (see Figure 10). Remove your two fingers and place this hand on top of your other hand. Interlock your fingers. Lean over the person with your arms straight and press down 4–5 cm (1.5–2 inches) (see Figure 11). Press 15 times and aim for a rate of 100 times per minute. Continue to deliver two breaths followed by 15 compressions until the ambulance service arrives.

key skills

Place the heel of one hand on the lower part of the breastbone. Place the other hand on top, interlock the fingers of both hands and compress the chest 4–5 cm (1.5–2 inches).

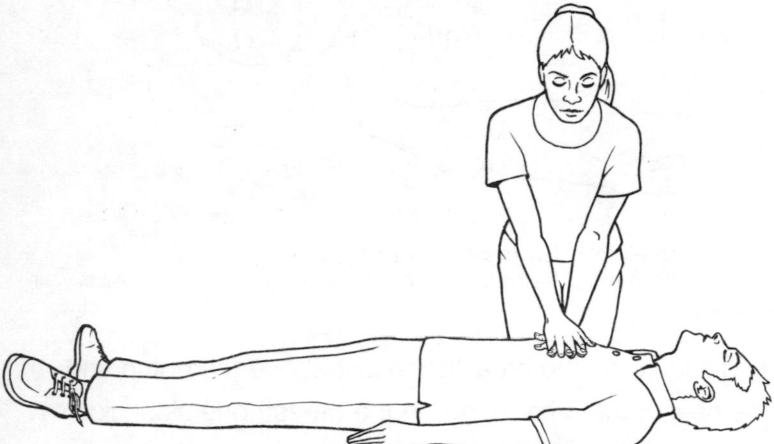

Fig 11 Keeping your arms straight, press down on the heel of your hands.

The combination of rescue breaths and chest compressions is known as 'Cardio Pulmonary Resuscitation' or CPR. Delivering CPR cannot only be an emotional and stressful experience, it can also be physically demanding. Even the fittest and most experienced people have reported how demanding it is to carry out CPR while waiting for the ambulance to arrive. However, we suggest that you only stop CPR when the ambulance personnel are in a position to take over or if you are suffering from fatigue and you are really unable to continue. Please remember that if there is a bystander who has the skills to carry out CPR, take turns. Throughout this whole procedure you must realize that your efforts are giving the person a chance of survival.

***one-minute** wonder*

Q Will I restart the heart by doing chest compressions?

A This is unlikely. To restart the heart, you need a machine that sends an electrical charge across the heart to try to restart it. This machine is called a defibrillator. However, by doing chest compressions, you are maintaining some blood circulation while waiting for the emergency services to bring the defibrillator.

summary

- For the unconscious person who is breathing, place him in the recovery position and call for an ambulance.
- For the unconscious person who is not breathing call for an ambulance and commence resuscitation.
- Remember to make sure that you, or someone else, has called for an ambulance before commencing CPR.

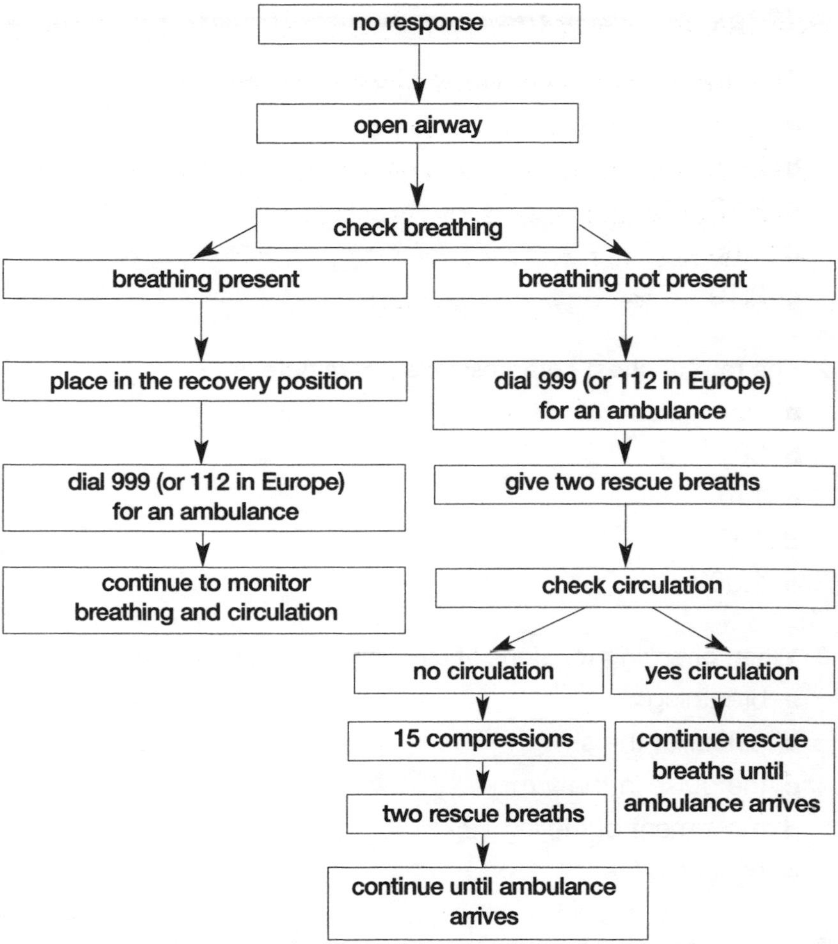

Assessing an unconscious person

self-testers

1 The ratio of rescue breaths to chest compressions is:

a 1:5
b 2:15
c 3:12
d 5:50
e 2:10

2 The rate of chest compressions per minute is:

a 50
b 80
c 140
d 100
e 1,000

3 When checking for signs of circulation you should look for:

a breathing
b colour of the skin
c the pulse in the arm
d movement of the leg
e coughing

4 You should place an unconscious person in the recovery position because:

a it is the most comfortable position to rest in
b it ensures the airway stays open
c if the person is sick, the vomit will drain away
d the tongue does not drop into the back of the throat
e the person may become violent

answers

1 **b**

2 **d**

3 **a**, **d** and **e**

4 **b**, **c** and **d**

3

choking

Choking is one of the more common situations that can become serious if you do not act quickly. Choking incidents involving adults tend to happen in public or when eating with family or friends, as most choking incidents involve food. What tends to happen is that some food falls to the back of the throat, which causes a muscular spasm (gagging). This results in the person trying to cough and breathe. In some cases the choking person tends to try and stifle the coughing because of embarrassment and this can make the situation worse. If the airway becomes completely blocked by a piece of food or foreign object the person will find it difficult to speak or breathe.

how to treat choking

You should start by encouraging the person to cough. Do this in a reassuring, rather than panicky, manner. If this does not work, get the person to lean forward. Support the person's chest with one hand and with the other hand give him up to five sharp slaps on the back between the shoulder blades. We say 'up to' five slaps because if the object becomes dislodged after one or two slaps there is no need to continue with the remaining slaps. It is important that these slaps are quite firm because you are attempting to create a vibration in the chest, which will hopefully move the object. Some people express concern about slapping the person too hard and hurting him but the risk of doing this is very slim. In fact, in our experience, the main reason why back slaps sometimes don't work is because they have not been delivered with sufficient force. After you have given the five back slaps you should check in the mouth just in case the object has come up into the mouth and you have not noticed.

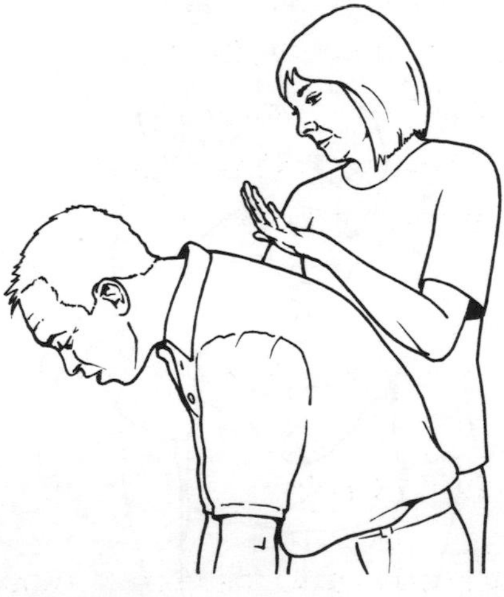

Fig 12 Treating a choking person – back slaps
Give up to five back slaps using the heel of the hand.

abdominal thrusts

If the five back slaps do not work, you should try abdominal thrusts. This procedure is also known as the the Heimlich manoeuvre. Stand behind the person who is choking, put your arms around his stomach, make a fist and grab your fist with your other hand. Position the fist on the abdomen between the ribs and underneath the breastbone. Pull inwards and upwards up to five times. Check in the mouth again to see if the object has become dislodged. If the object has not moved, repeat the back slaps and abdominal thrusts up to three more times if necessary. Then call for an ambulance.

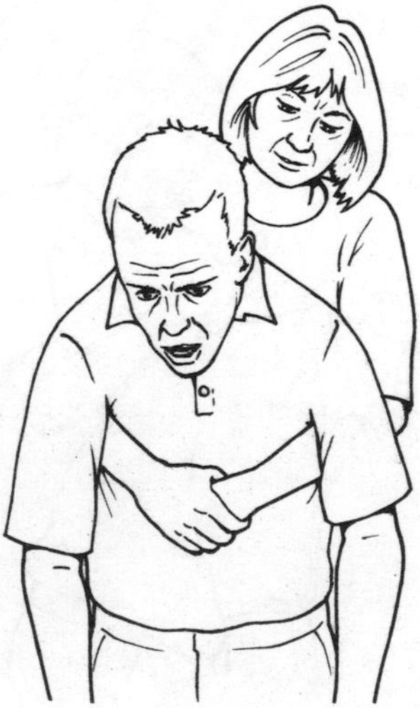

Fig 13 Treating a choking person – abdominal thrusts
Pull inwards and upwards up to five times.

> ***one-minute** wonder*
>
> **Q** Is the abdominal thrust a way of making the person cough?
>
> **A** No, the aim of the abdominal thrust is to push air from the lungs at high speed up the windpipe in an attempt to dislodge the blockage.

If, at any stage, the person stops breathing and becomes unconscious, you must try to give rescue breaths. If it is not possible to get air into the person using rescue breaths (you will feel resistance to the air and the person's chest will not rise and fall), then commence chest compressions as these may help to dislodge the object (see Chapter 2, page 24).

> ***one-minute** wonder*
>
> **Q** Are the chest compressions for choking the same as the ones described for CPR?
>
> **A** The technique is exactly the same, but, the purpose of doing them is different. In the choking situation the purpose is to dislodge the blockage.

> ***one-minute** wonder*
>
> **Q** Is it possible to perform abdominal thrusts without removing the person's clothes?
>
> **A** Yes, removing clothing is not necessary and trying to remove it will only delay the care.

key skills

To treat a choking adult:

- you should encourage the person to cough
- give up to five back slaps
- give up to five abdominal thrusts
- repeat if necessary
- if the blockage does not clear, give the back slaps and abdominal thrusts three times and then call an ambulance.
- if the person becomes unconscious call an ambulance.

summary

The main thing to remember when dealing with a situation such as choking is to take control. Give back slaps and abdominal thrusts if necessary. If the person collapses be prepared to resuscitate and call for an ambulance.

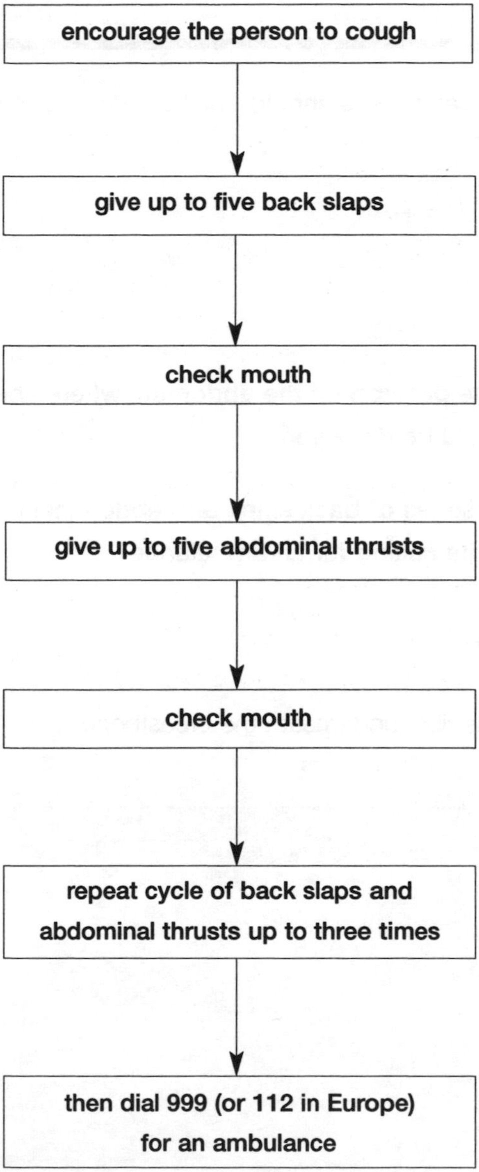
encourage the person to cough
give up to five back slaps
check mouth
give up to five abdominal thrusts
check mouth
repeat cycle of back slaps and abdominal thrusts up to three times
then dial 999 (or 112 in Europe) for an ambulance

How to treat choking

self-testers

1 How many back slaps should you initially give to a choking person?

a 5

b 10

c 15

d 12

2 Describe the position on the abdomen, where abdominal thrusts should be delivered.

3 How many series of back slaps and abdominal thrusts should you do before calling for an ambulance?

---

answers

1 **a**

2 between the ribs, underneath the breastbone

3 **3**

4

5 minute first aid

severe bleeding

The average adult has 8 pints (5 litres) of blood in their body. In our experience, severe bleeding, if untreated, can result in shock and, in a small number of cases, this can prove fatal. It is possible to lose up to 25 per cent of your blood volume without the situation becoming critical, so in the average adult this equates to 2 pints (1¼ litres) of blood. If you are concerned that a person is suffering from severe blood loss, your prompt action can ensure that the situation does not deteriorate and may contribute to a significant improvement in the person's condition.

bleeding

If bleeding is severe it can be dramatic and distressing, especially if there is a large wound somewhere on the body that is causing the bleeding. In this chapter we will focus on severe blood loss.

The severity of the bleeding from the wound depends on the location, size and depth of the wound. Some parts of the body appear to bleed heavily, when in fact the actual blood loss is not significant. This applies particularly to the scalp, which has a large network of small blood vessels, so that even if there is just a small cut to the scalp, there may appear to be a large blood loss. On the other hand, a very small tear of the vein in somebody who suffers from varicose veins will lead to copious blood loss, and this may be life threatening if not properly and promptly treated. We will focus on blood loss outside the body but it is also worth remembering that internal bleeding may also occur without any sign of blood.

When treating a severe bleed, your aims are to:

- stop the bleeding as quickly as possible
- prevent the onset of shock
- minimize the risk of infection.

To stop the bleeding, quickly place pressure directly on the wound using your hand, the person's own hand or a clean pad, if available. At the same time, raise the injured limb above the level of the heart. This helps to reduce the blood flow to the wound by using gravity and ensuring that all the essential organs are kept adequately supplied with blood. In the event of a leg wound, it is important to help the person to lie down and elevate the leg above the level of the heart. If the injury is on the arm, the person should sit down and elevate the arm. Once the limb is elevated, secure a pad or dressing in place, ensuring that pressure is maintained.

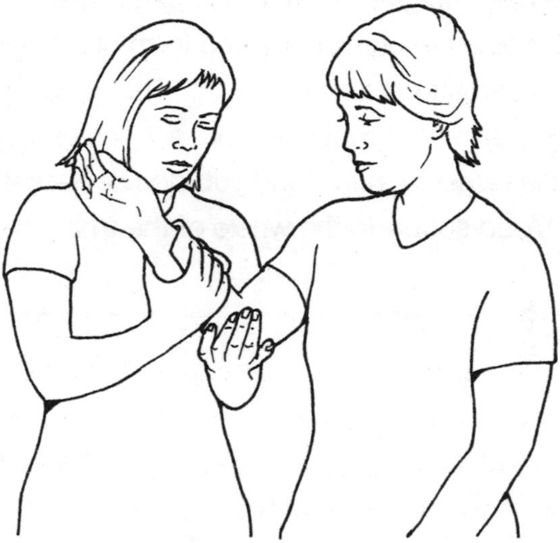

Fig 14 Treating a severe bleed
Hold the dressing firmly over the wound.

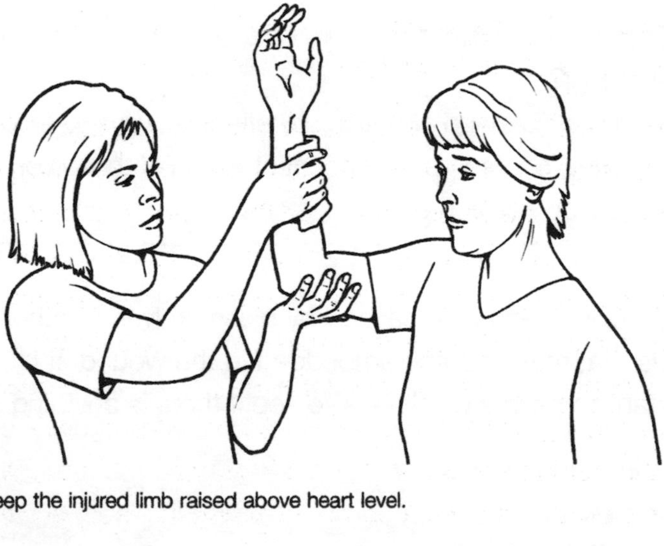

Fig 15 Keep the injured limb raised above heart level.

You may have been taught if you are caring for a severe bleed that you should apply a tourniquet in the form of a tie or a narrow piece of clothing around the affected limb. This is no longer a recommended first-aid procedure because it has been proven that to stem the blood to the wound you do not necessarily have to cut off the blood supply to the whole of the limb.

key skills

To treat a major bleed:

- apply pressure to the wound
- if the wound is on a limb elevate it above the level of the heart
- call for an ambulance and continue to reassure the person.

one-minute wonder

Q Should I apply direct pressure on the wound first or should I elevate it?

A Both pressure and elevation are effective ways to stop the bleeding, and so it's not important which of these you do first so long as you do both.

Many severe bleeds are caused by glass, knives or other sharp objects that may become embedded in the wound. It is important to have a quick look to see if there is anything embedded in the wound. If there is an object embedded in the wound you should not remove it as it may be helping to stem the blood flow and by removing it you may increase the blood loss and cause further internal damage. To treat a wound with an embedded object you should apply pressure to the edges of the wound and bandage around the object ensuring you do not apply direct pressure to it. If there is an embedded object ensure that the person receives immediate medical attention as the object will need to be removed in a surgical procedure and the resulting wound treated accordingly.

5 • 5

shock

Shock is a term used to describe a range of situations from feeling very anxious about the bleeding incident to a serious clinical state that occurs as a result of a loss of blood from the body's circulation. The loss of a lot of blood from the body is referred to as clinical shock and can be life threatening because the vital organs (such as the brain, heart and kidneys) are not getting enough blood for them to function properly.

how to recognize clinical shock

In a case of clinical shock there will be an injury that is causing the blood loss. In addition to this the person will have pale, cold and clammy skin, a rapid and weak pulse, and fast and shallow breathing. The person will feel restless, thirsty and nauseated and may actually vomit. If the bleeding is not stopped and the state of clinical shock worsens, then the person will gradually lose consciousness and the condition becomes life threatening. It is therefore important to recognize clinical shock and try to do something about it as soon as you can.

treating shock

It is important to treat the underlying problem as soon as possible. Help the person to lie down and raise the legs above the level of the heart so that the blood in the legs flows towards the centre of the body where it is most needed. Keep the person warm by covering him with a light blanket and make constant reassurances, as the person will feel anxious. As soon as you have recognized that a person is suffering from clinical shock, you must call the emergency services.

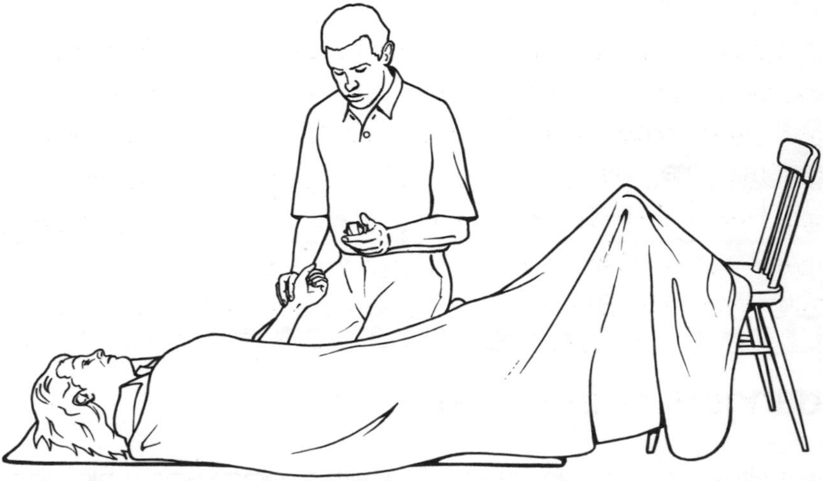

Fig 16 In the case of shock raise the person's legs as high as possible.

one-minute wonder

Q My mother told me that you should always make the person in shock sit down and give them a sweet cup of tea and a stiff drink. Is this wise?

A There is no clinical evidence to support drinking tea or alcohol. We recommend that a person in shock has nothing to eat, drink or smoke until they have been seen in hospital.

key skills

To treat shock you should:

- treat the cause
- call for an ambulance
- raise the legs
- keep the person warm.

dangers of infection

In a situation where you are dealing with a person who is bleeding, there is a potential risk of transferring infectious organisms such as viruses and bacteria from one person to another. Therefore, it is wise to take some simple precautions such as wearing disposable gloves (if they are available) and using the person's hand rather than yours to apply pressure on a bleeding wound. Try to avoid splashing blood into your eyes or mouth and use a plastic bag to dispose of any blood-stained rubbish.

one-minute wonder

Q If I do not have gloves, what should I do?

A If you do not have gloves, you must not hold back from life-saving procedures but you can cover your hands with clean plastic bags and make sure that if you have any wounds on your hands they are covered with waterproof dressings.

summary

We know the sight of blood is off-putting for most people, and seeing a lot of blood often gives the impression of a severe injury – this is not always the case.

- If there is damage to a major blood vessel and you do not apply direct pressure and elevation the person can go into shock.
- Bleeding is one of the conditions where basic first-aid skills (elevation and pressure) can prevent the situation getting worse and may well improve the person's condition.

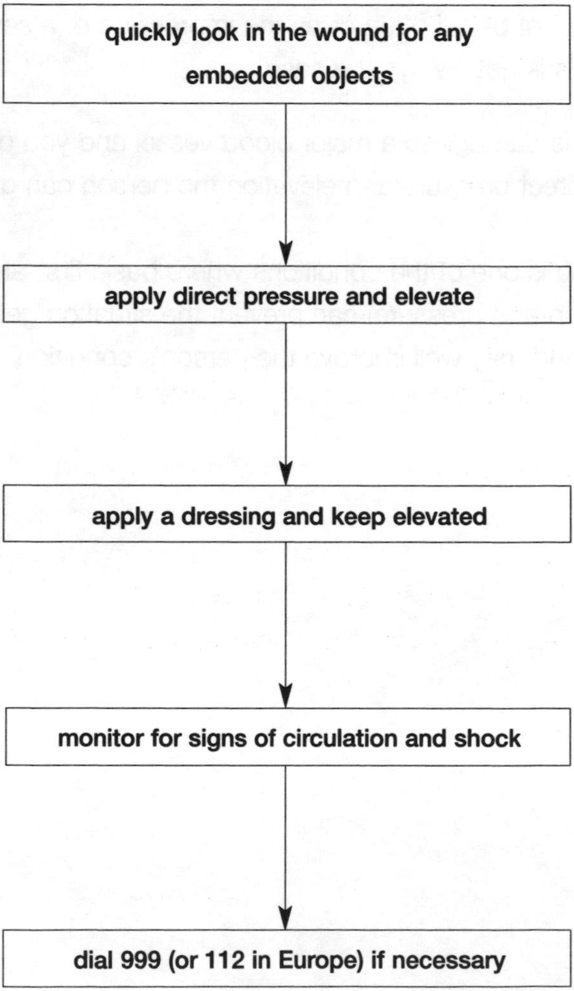

How to treat a severe bleed

self-testers

1 The treatment for a serious bleed is:

a apply pressure and elevate

b tie a tourniquet

c pour water on it

2 In the event of a conscious person going into shock, you should:

a give the person alcohol

b keep the person warm

c lie the person down

d put the person in the recovery position

3 If there is a piece of glass in a wound you should:

a remove it slowly and elevate

b remove it quickly in the direction it went into the wound

c leave it in place and dress around it

d apply a dressing over the object without moving it

answers

1 **a**

2 **b** and **c**

3 **c**

5

common emergency situations

In this chapter we will look at some of the more common emergency situations you may encounter. We recognize that each situation presents a unique problem, and specific management will depend on the location of the incident, the number of injured people and the type of injuries the people have. Therefore although it is not possible to be definitive in the advice we offer, we can highlight the key things you should do and some of the things you should not do in these situations.

In the previous chapters we have reinforced the importance of you as the first aider not taking unacceptable risks to help someone. It is worth mentioning that there may be some situations in which it may be too dangerous for you to help and the only first-aid action you can carry out is making a call to the emergency services.

5

fire

If you are inside a burning building your priority is the same as in any other emergency – to ensure the safety of yourself and others with you. Raise the alarm, by either activating the fire alarm if there is one nearby or shouting for help. It is also important to call the emergency services. Most public buildings have dedicated fire wardens and it is important to follow their advice. In the event of a fire in any building, you must not attempt to fight the fire unless you are familiar with how to use fire-fighting equipment and have already called the emergency services.

You should leave the building as quickly as possible but in an orderly manner. People naturally tend to panic in a fire situation so it is important that you as a first aider demonstrate a calmness and an authority that will be reassuring to the other people involved. If the fire is in a public building such as a place of work you should be aware of the evacuation procedure and the escape route. Most work places have a dedicated assembly point, ensure you know where this is. If the fire is in your home you may want to think about how you would escape. It's a good idea to plan an escape route from each room in the house.

You should never attempt to re-enter a building once you have escaped – forget about your coat, handbag and your credit cards as you can replace them if they are damaged. If there is a lot of smoke as you escape or if you are trapped in a smoke-filled building remember to keep as close to the floor as possible as this is where the air is cleanest. If you or someone you are caring for has inhaled a quantity of smoke or you suspect they may have, you should seek medical advice.

If you are in a car and there is evidence or a risk of fire you should stop the car in a safe place. Switch off the engine. Get out of the vehicle and evacuate any passengers. Only attempt to fight the fire if it's small and you have a fire extinguisher. Warn any bystanders to move away in case the vehicle explodes.

To treat burns cool the area under cold running water for at least ten minutes and cover with a clean non-fluffy pad or clingfilm. Call for an ambulance or take the people to hospital.

key skills

In a fire situation:

- stay calm
- raise the alarm
- follow the evacuation procedure.

***one-minute** wonder*

Q You often see people on TV and in the movies putting handkerchiefs over their mouths to avoid inhaling smoke. Does this work?

A It can help a little, but it will only filter out a small amount of the smoke. Remember the handkerchief has to be made of linen or a similiar material, a tissue does not work.

5 • 5

clothes on fire

If you come across a fire situation in which a person's clothing is on fire you should follow the **Stop**, **Drop**, **Wrap** and **Roll** technique:

- **Stop** – Don't let the person run around as the movement of air will fan the flames and increase the burning.
- **Drop** – Get the person to drop onto the ground. If you have to assist the person to lay down be careful not to get burned.
- **Wrap** – Cover the person in a blanket, thick coat or in a heavy fabric like a rug.
- **Roll** – Roll the person on the ground until the flames have been extinguished.

key skills

To assist someone whose clothes are on fire, remember **Stop**, **Drop**, **Wrap** and **Roll**.

road traffic accident

On the arrival at the scene of a road traffic accident, your immediate concern should be to secure the scene so that a second accident does not occur. If you are in a car, park it safely, a little way back from the accident with your hazard warning lights on. Try and make sure other road users can see you by wearing a reflective jacket or light-coloured clothing if possible. Try and identify the number of injured people involved and the seriousness of their injuries. Remember the DRABC you read about in Chapter 1 as part of the assessment. Call the emergency services and try and give them as much information as possible about those involved. Try and be as accurate as possible about the location. Think about the emergency services you require – in the case of a traffic accident where there is an injured person you are advised to call the police as well as the ambulance service. If there is a spillage of fuel or chemicals involved, or if there is someone trapped in a vehicle, you may require the fire service as well. Briefly survey the scene and position of the vehicles. Was it a high- or low-speed accident?

Was it a side collision or a rear shunt? These observations may give you useful information about the kind or severity of the injuries you have to deal with.

In the event of coming across an accident involving a motorcyclist, the question of whether to remove the injured person's helmet or not presents a real dilemma for many first aiders. The advice, in its simplest form, is as follows. If, on assessing the person, you do not get a response, it can be very difficult to assess the airway and breathing with the helmet on, therefore you have no choice other than to gently remove it. Continue the ABC check and respond accordingly. However, if the person talks to you during assessment there is no need to remove the helmet. Leave the person in the position he is in and treat any life-threatening injuries he may have. Continue to talk to the person and monitor his condition until the ambulance arrives.

***one-minute** wonder*

Q I read in a book that if you attend an accident and there is more than one person injured, you should ignore the person who is calling out in pain and go to the one who is quiet. Is this true and if so, why?

A It is not a good idea to ignore any injured person, but the point you make is correct. A person who is able to call out is obviously conscious and while this person's injuries may be serious, priority should always be given to an unconscious person.

key skills

If you attend a road traffic accident:

- you should ensure your own safety
- find out the number and condition of the injured people
- call the emergency services
- perform life-saving first aid.

electrical injuries in the home

The popularity of DIY has significantly increased the number of electricity-related injuries in the home, many of which result from enthusiasts drilling or hammering screws or nails into live circuits. Other electricity-related injuries are a result of householders attempting repairs while the electrical current is still on. Electrical injuries are also caused by adults taking electrical appliances into the bathroom. Gardening accidents involving mowers and hedge trimmers are also common electrical accidents.

Many electricity-related accidents would not occur if the user were to take simple precautions such as ensuring the current is switched off before working with electric components, using a circuit breaker with tools and electrical gardening equipment, and never touching sockets or switches with wet hands.

On approaching the scene of a possible electrocution, you should switch off the current before you touch the injured person. If you touch the person while he is still in contact with the current you could also receive an electric shock. If you cannot switch off the current you should try and remove the cable from the the part of the person's body that is touching the cable. You can do this by standing on something dry like a telephone directory and then using something wooden, like a broom handle, to move the cable away from the person. Do not use anything metallic as this will conduct electricity. Once it is safe to do so, carry out the ABC check (see Chapter 1).

drowning

Many drowning incidents result from people swimming in cold water or in water with strong currents. Other such incidents occur when people over-estimate their fitness or swimming ability and some people die as a result of swimming under the influence of alcohol and drugs.

In a drowning situation your priority as a first aider is to get the person out of the water as quickly as possible so that you can assess his condition. If possible try and reach the person from dry land using a stick or a rope. Only enter the water to rescue a person if you are a trained lifesaver. On getting the person out of the water, carry him with his head lower than his chest. This allows any water to drain out and keeps the airway clear if he vomits. If you are unable to carry the person, drag him to dry ground and assess his condition. Because of the temperature of the water, near-drowning victims are at risk from hypothermia. Therefore once the person has been removed from the water, lay him on a blanket or coat and cover him with whatever clothing you have got available. Check the ABC (see Chapter 1) and call for an ambulance.

heart attack

A heart attack occurs as a result of a blockage in the blood supply to the muscle of the heart. The severity of the attack depends on how much of the muscle is affected. The larger the area affected, the greater the risk to the person. Many heart attack victims show signs of difficulty in breathing and have severe pain in the centre of the chest (this pain can affect one or both of the arms and sometimes radiates up to the jaw or through to the back). The person will also appear sweaty and pale, often with a blue tinge around the earlobes and lips. Your first objective as a first aider is to make the person comfortable by sitting him in the position shown in Figure 17. Then call for an ambulance and tell the call handler that you suspect the person has had a heart attack – this will allow the ambulance to give the call the highest priority. If the person is conscious give him a 300 mg tablet of aspirin to chew – this may help to prevent the blood clot increasing in size and will help with the person's recovery. Continue to reassure the person until the ambulance arrives. Remember to tell the ambulance crew you have given the person aspirin.

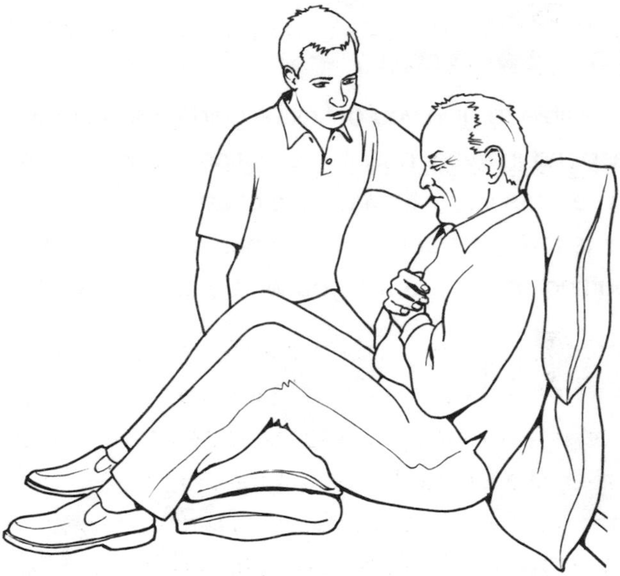

Fig 17 In the case of a heart attack, sit the person down, make him comfortable, and reassure him.

***one-minute** wonder*

Q If I do not have aspirin, will a paracetamol do?

A No, paracetamol does not work in the same way as aspirin and will not help the person's recovery.

key skills

If you suspect a person is having a heart attack:

- sit the person down
- call an ambulance
- give an aspirin
- reassure the person.

summary

It is not possible to give you definitive guidance on how you should respond in every possible situation. As we say, each scenario presents you with a unique challenge. The key thing to remember is that your actions can make a difference but if you end up putting yourself at risk you will be of little assistance.

self-testers

1 If a person's clothing is on fire, what should you do? (Remember SDWR.)

2 Which of the following is not a typical sign of a heart attack?

a severe chest pain
b hot and dry skin
c pain in the arms
d shortage of breath

3 Which of the following can be safely used to move a live electric cable?

a a broom handle
b a metal clothes line prop
c an ironing board
d a vacuum cleaner attachment

4 On carrying a drowning victim from the water, the head should be:

a lower than the chest
b higher than the chest
c level with the chest
d level with the legs

answers

1 **S**top; **D**rop; **W**rap; **R**oll

2 **b**

3 **a**

4 **a**

case studies

Andrea's story

Andrea Brown didn't expect to have to use her life-saving skills when she entered a large distribution warehouse to carry out some training with the staff on how to move heavy and bulky goods. On her arrival she noticed that there was a lot of commotion at one of the entrance doors. A small group of employees had gathered and it was clear that all was not well as they were staring at the ground with concerned looks on their faces. 'It was really strange,' said Andrea, 'they were all obviously concerned but no one appeared to be doing anything.'

On arriving on the scene it was clear to Andrea that the person lying on the floor was unwell. He was 'deathly white and obviously unconscious'. He was not breathing and there were no signs of circulation. Andrea asked one of the bystanders to call for an ambulance and then she started CPR. Soon after she had started resuscitation the collapsed man began to vomit. She turned him onto his side to allow the vomit to drain out and then asked if there was a first-aid kit on the premises. There was a first-aid kit to hand but unfortunately it did not have a face shield in it. 'To be absolutely honest doing mouth-to-mouth on a person is quite off-putting but doing it on a person who had just been sick was horrible.' However, Andrea persevered, and the 12 minutes until the ambulance paramedics arrived seemed like a lifetime.

Some of the images of the incident that remain with Andrea concern the appearance of the person, 'I had never seen anyone look so pale and unwell.' As an avid viewer of hospital dramas on television Andrea thought she may have some insight into what it feels like to have to respond in an emergency situation, but it wasn't like this in real life. The thing that amazed her was that before the event she thought she was the type of person who would be too scared to step forward to help. When faced with the situation 'I just got some inner strength, belief and confidence from somewhere, you just feel you want to help.' On reflection, Andrea feels some anger about what happened, anger that some of the person's work colleagues were just 'standing around' not knowing what to do. She has asked herself many times since why nobody had called for an ambulance and she can only assume that the bystanders were in a state of shock, seeing one of their relatively young and healthy workmates lying on the ground.

Andrea is affected by the outcome of the incident. Unfortunately, the man involved in the incident died. Andrea has spoken to family and friends about what happened but cannot help but ask herself whether she could have done anything differently.

authors' observations

We think this is a very honest and realistic overview of what it really feels like to be involved in an attempt to resuscitate someone. The feeling of being 'unprepared' for an incident is very common – people with first-aid skills never know when they are going to be called upon to use them, and often it is when it is least expected. The idea that colleagues were observing what was going on yet nobody remembered to call for an ambulance concerned Andrea – she may be correct in thinking that they could have been shaken by what they had experienced. There's also the possibility that everyone thought somebody else had made the call to the emergency services, when in fact nobody had made the call. This is not uncommon and we often find that the larger the number of bystanders, the more likely it is for an individual to forget the basics like calling for an ambulance or checking to see if the person is breathing. This reads like a situation that needed someone with Andrea's authority to step forward and take charge, to make sure that key things were done as efficiently as possible.

Andrea spoke about the unpleasantness of giving rescue breaths – many people on leaving our first-aid courses feel like this. Rescue breathing tends to be top of the list of things people have reservations about doing. When faced with an emergency situation, especially if we know the person involved, we tend to find the inner strength to step forward and to carry out some of the more unpleasant and potentially life-saving aspects of first aid.

In an ideal situation there will be some basic equipment like a first-aid kit available, but many first-aid incidents occur in places where there is very little to work with. In Andrea's case it would have been helpful to have had a face shield when the person started being sick. There are various types of face shield available on the market, usually made of plastic or polythene. These products provide a barrier between a first aider and the person, ensuring better hygiene and reducing the risk of cross infection. We must point out that performing rescue breathing without one of these devices presents a very small risk of infection to you or the other person, but not having one available must not be a deterrent to attempting rescue breathing.

The outcome of this incident left Andrea wondering whether she had done everything she could to save this person's life. The outcome was sad but the most important thing was that Andrea did what she could to help and gave the person a chance.

Graham's story

A family treat to celebrate Graham Elliot's birthday turned into a night he would never forget. His wife and children had gone to great efforts to keep the dinner date at a posh local restaurant a secret from him. There was a look of genuine surprise on his face when he arrived to find his extended family and friends occupying most of the restaurant tables.

Fish was the speciality at this particular restaurant, and Graham had a delicious seafood starter followed by the chef's special, described on the menu as 'a pick-and-mix of the best our sea waters have to offer'. Graham plumped for this, as white fish was a particular favourite of his.

The sudden 'scratching' Graham felt in his throat was obviously as a result of swallowing a fish bone. At first he tried to avoid drawing attention to himself by stifling his coughs, which were more like gasps, behind his 'cleanly-laundered napkin'. His wife was sitting next to him and, while aware of his muffled coughs, had no idea that he was choking. His wife told him to have a drink of water. The water did not help and Graham seriously began to panic. The diner next to him told him to eat a piece of the bread roll that was on his side plate to push the object down. This clearly made the situation worse and Graham now began to have difficulty breathing and had managed to grab the attention of most of the diners and waiters in the restaurant.

Graham's brother-in-law started slapping him on the back but this did not appear to have any effect. Graham was now feeling sick, frightened and embarrassed. Graham then began to feel faint and dizzy and he felt like he was being strangled.

Then, suddenly, the soggy lump of bread came back out of his mouth and he felt that he was able to breathe again. He was still in pain and experiencing a burning sensation at the back of his mouth and in his throat. His daughter took him to hospital and on examination the small fish bone was still stuck in his throat. He had to have an operation to have the bone removed under anaesthetic. Graham was discharged from hospital three days later and even now, two years later, he still feels guilty about spoiling everyone's night out.

authors' observations

You get a real sense of Graham's panic and distress from reading this story. The actions of Graham's brother-in-law who gave the back slaps probably saved him from becoming unconscious.

If back slaps had been combined with abdominal thrusts, they may have helped to dislodge the blockage. Clearly, giving the person bread to swallow in an attempt to move the object was not a good idea – it probably contributed to Graham being unable to breathe. Fish bones can be dangerous if they become stuck in the throat, but they do not tend to inhibit breathing. Sufficient air can usually pass the bone to enable the person to breathe. However, the damage the bone causes to the back of the throat can cause the soft tissue to swell and impact on the choking person's ability to breathe. Choking incidents involving fish bones should always be checked out in hospital if they result in painful throats, to ensure the bone is no longer present and to check if there is swelling of the soft tissue.

Raj's story

Raj Khan was no stranger to using knives – he came from a long line of butchers and followed in the family tradition. It was therefore ironic that the only serious knife-related injury he suffered was while he was at home preparing food for a family banquet.

'In the butchering world it is said that the knife is an extension of your hand', says Raj. 'I was using tools I was not familiar with and filleting fish can be tricky.' However, this wasn't just a trivial case of a workman blaming his tools, as the outcome of the knife slipping was much more serious than that. The blade only made a shallow, clean cut to his wrist but the blood appeared quickly and profusely. There was blood all over the work surface and the floor. Raj was very surprised that it was not painful. He quickly tied a tea towel around the cut in his wrist. The blood quickly began to soak through the tea towel. Raj removed the original towel and replaced it with a clean one but at this point he began to feel unwell. Thankfully his brother arrived at this point and as he had some first-aid knowledge he held the tea towel in place and helped his brother to lie on the sofa. He helped keep the injured wrist above the level of the heart but this was not easy as Raj was obviously unwell and appeared to faint. Raj's brother kept the hand elevated while he called for an ambulance. On arrival, the ambulance crew set up a drip as Raj had lost so much blood, and they took him to hospital. The wound was cleaned and stitched in hospital. Raj was kept in overnight for observations and discharged the next day.

authors' observations

Some people under-estimate the amount of blood that can be lost from a relatively small wound. The area around the wrist is particularly at risk as in this area some large blood vessels run very close to the surface of the skin and can be damaged by shallow cuts. Raj's observation that he had lost a lot of blood was probably true, but the scene in the kitchen may have looked worse because the blood was falling on lightly-coloured non-absorbent surfaces.

Raj did quite a good job of administering first aid to himself, however one of the difficulties he probably faced was applying pressure to the wound with the tea towel. It would have been more effective if he had raised his arm above the level of the heart and used the tea towel as a pad once it was elevated. Removing the first tea towel was not a good idea as the blood may have begun to clot and removing the tea towel could have restarted the bleeding. It would have been preferable to apply the second tea towel over the first one. Laying Raj down on the sofa was a good idea, however, if the sofa was a significant distance from the kitchen it may have been better to lay him on the kitchen floor. You should avoid walking a person who is already unsteady on his feet.

first-aid kit contents

There are no hard and fast rules about what should be in your personal first-aid kit. What you're most likely to need will depend on where you are and what you're doing. You may wish to keep a kit at home, another in your car and perhaps a small version to take with you on holidays, etc. What is vital is that you have the supplies you need ready to hand for when you need them.

There are some core items that we recommend you have in any kit:

- **plasters in assorted sizes** – these are applied to small cuts and grazes. Covering the wound with a clean, dry dressing will help prevent the area from becoming infected as well as help to stop any bleeding.
- **sterile wound dressings in assorted sizes** – these are used for wounds such as cuts or burns. Place the dressing pad over the injured area, making sure that the pad is larger than the wound. Then wrap the roller bandage around the limb to secure it.
- **triangular bandages** – commonly used for slings, these are strong supportive bandages. If they are sterile then they can also be used as dressings for wounds and burns.
- **safety pins** – useful for securing crêpe bandages and triangular bandages.

- **adhesive tape** – useful to hold and secure bandages comfortably in place. Some people are allergic to the adhesive, but hypoallergenic tape is available.
- **sterile gauze swabs** – these can be used to clean around a wound or in conjunction with other bandages and tape to help keep wounds clean and dry.
- **non-alcoholic cleansing wipes** – useful for cleaning cuts and grazes. They can also be used to clean your hands if water and soap are not available.
- **roller bandages** – used to give support to injured joints, to secure dressings in place, to maintain pressure on them, and to limit swelling.
- **disposable gloves** – these single-use gloves are an important safety measure to avoid infecting wounds as well as to protect you.
- **scissors** – using a round-ended pair of scissors will not cause injury and will make short work of cutting dressings or bandages to size. It is useful to have a strong pair that will cut through clothing.
- **burn gel** – use directly on a burn to cool and relieve the pain of minor burns and to help prevent infection. Very useful if water is not available.
- **ice pack** – cooling an injury and the surrounding area can reduce swelling and pain. Always wrap an ice pack in a dry cloth and do not use it for more than ten minutes at one application.
- **tweezers** – useful for picking out splinters.
- **thermometer** – used to assess the body temperature. There

are several different types including the traditional glass mercury thermometer and digital thermometer, as well as the forehead thermometer and the ear sensor. Normal body temperature is 37°C.

- **face shield or pocket mask** (a hygiene shield for giving rescue breaths) – these are plastic barriers with a reinforced hole to fit over the injured person's mouth. Use the shield to protect you and the injured person from infections when giving rescue breaths.
- **note pad and pen** – use the pad to record any information about the injured person that may be of use to the emergency services when they arrive. For example, the name and address of the person, how the accident occurred, and any observations. It is also useful to record vital signs so that you can monitor how well the person is doing over a period of time.
- **basic first-aid information** – a basic guide to first-aid tips, and emergency information (you can use the first aid essentials pull-out card in this book).

This is not an exhaustive list and there are many more items you may find useful to add to your kit, such as antiseptic cream, but remember that after the product has been opened it is no longer sterile.

It's easy to make your own first-aid kit by collecting these items or, alternatively, you could simply buy a complete kit. For more information on British Red Cross kits go to **www.redcross.org.uk/firstaidproducts** or call 0845 601 7105.

The Health and Safety Executive (HSE) is responsible for the regulation of almost all the risks to health and safety arising from work activity in Britain. Regulations concerning kit contents apply to employers. For more information about first-aid kits and training for the workplace go to **www.redcrossfirstaidtraining.co.uk** or call 0870 170 9110.

household first-aid equipment

Throughout this book we have made reference to the importance of having first-aid skills, knowledge and equipment. In terms of equipment, we recommend you have a well-stocked first-aid kit (see page 71), but we also recognize that there are emergency situations where you will not have access to any of the equipment. In such situations you will have to be creative and use whatever equipment is available to you. In this section we have identified some of the items most of us already have in our homes and suggest how they can be useful in a first-aid situation.

- **beer** – you may not always have access to cold running water when treating a burn or scald. In this case, use some other cold liquid like beer, soft drink or milk. The aim is to cool the burnt area as quickly as possible using whatever cold liquid is available. Beer can be used to cool the area while waiting for water or while walking the person to a supply of cold running water. Remember, the area should be cooled for at least ten minutes for the treatment to be effective.
- **chair** – a chair has numerous first-aid uses; when treating a nosebleed, sit the person down while pinching the nose and tilting the head forward. If you are treating a bleed from a large wound to the leg, you should lay the person down and raise the leg above the level of the heart. A chair is ideal for this purpose.

- **chocolate** – chocolate can be given to a conscious person who is diabetic and having a hypoglycaemia attack known as a "hypo". This can help raise the person's blood sugar. Chocolate can also be given to a person with hypothermia as high-energy foods will help to warm the person up.
- **cling film** – cling film can be used to wrap around a burn or a scald once it has cooled. It is an ideal covering as it does not stick to the burn. It also keeps the burnt area clean and because it is transparent, you can continue to monitor the burn without removing the covering.
- **credit card** – when an insect sting is visible on the skin, a credit card can be used to scrape it away. Using the edge of the credit card, drag it across the skin. This will remove the sting. Using a credit card is preferable to using a pair of tweezers as some stings contain a sac of poison and if the sting is grasped with tweezers you may inject the sac of poison into the skin. If you do not have a credit card you can use the back of a kitchen knife or any other object similar to a credit card.
- **food bag** – a clean freezer or sandwich bag makes an ideal cover for a burn or scald to the hand. The injured part should be placed in the bag once the cooling has finished. By placing it in the bag you reduce the risk of infection and it also helps reduce the level of pain.
- **frozen peas** – frozen peas or other frozen small fruit and vegetables can be used to treat a sprain or strain. Wrap the peas in a tea towel or something similar and place them onto

the injury. This will help to reduce pain and swelling. Peas are ideal as they can be moulded around the injury more easily than bigger fruit and vegetables.

- **milk** – if an adult tooth is dislodged and cannot be placed back in its socket, it should be placed in a container of milk. This will stop it drying out and increase the possibility of it being successfully replanted by a dental surgeon.
- **paper bag** – a panic attack often results in the person hyperventilating (breathing very quickly). Reassure the person and get them to breath into a paper bag, this will help to regulate and slow down the persons breathing.
- **steam** – if your child has an attack of croup, sit your child on your knee in the bathroom. Run the tap to create a steamy atmosphere, this may help to relieve the symptoms.
- **vinegar** – if a person is stung by a tropical jellyfish, pour vinegar over the site of the sting. This will help to stop the poison spreading around the body.
- **water** – cold running water is the preferred treatment for burns and scalds. Place the burn under a cold water tap as quickly as possible and leave it there for at least ten minutes.
- **Yellow Pages and a broom** – in the event of having to provide assistance to a person with an electrical injury, where the person is attached to the current, you can stand on a copy of the Yellow Pages to insulate yourself from an electrical shock. You should then move the electrical cable away using a dry piece of wood, a broom handle is ideal.

about the Red Cross

the British Red Cross and the International Red Cross and Red Crescent Movement

The British Red Cross is a leading UK charity with 40,000 volunteers working in almost every community. We provide a range of high-quality services in local communities across the UK every day. We respond to emergencies, train first aiders, help vulnerable people regain their independence, and assist refugees and asylum seekers.

The British Red Cross is part of the International Red Cross and Red Crescent Movement, the world's largest independent humanitarian organization. This Movement comprises three components: the International Committee of the Red Cross; the International Federation of Red Cross and Red Crescent Societies; and 181 National Red Cross and National Red Crescent Societies around the world.

As a member of the International Red Cross and Red Crescent Movement, the British Red Cross is committed to, and bound by, its Fundamental Principles:

- Humanity
- Impartiality
- Neutrality
- Independence
- Voluntary Service
- Unity
- Universality.

the International Committee of the Red Cross

Based in Geneva, Switzerland, the International Committee of the Red Cross (ICRC) is a private, independent humanitarian institution, whose role is defined as part of the Geneva Conventions. Serving as a neutral intermediary during international wars and civil conflicts, it provides protection and assistance for civilians, prisoners of war and the wounded, and provides a similar function during internal disturbances.

To find out more visit **www.icrc.org**

the International Federation of Red Cross and Red Crescent Societies

Also based in Geneva, the Federation is a separately constituted body that co-ordinates international relief provided by National Societies for victims of natural disasters, and for refugees and displaced persons outside conflict zones. It also assists Red Cross and Red Crescent Societies with their own development, helping them to plan and implement disaster preparedness and development projects on behalf of vulnerable people in local communities.

To find out more visit **www.ifrc.org**

National Red Cross and National Red Crescent Societies

In most countries around the world, there exists a National Red Cross or Red Crescent Society. Each Society has a responsibility to help vulnerable people within its own borders, and to work in conjunction with the Movement to protect and support those in crisis worldwide.

To find out more about the British Red Cross, visit **www.redcross.org.uk**

useful addresses

NHS Direct

www.nhsdirect.nhs.uk

Tel: 0845 46 47 (24 hours)

Preparing for Emergencies – Government Advice

www.preparingforemergencies.gov.uk

Tel: 0800 88 77 77

Textphone: 08000 859 859

The Royal Life Saving Society UK

www.lifesavers.org.uk

Lifesavers, River House, High Street, Broom, Warwickshire, B50 4HN

Tel: 01789 773994

Fax: 01789 773995

E-mail: lifesavers@rlss.org.uk

International Red Cross contact details

Australia

National Office, 155 Pelham Street, 3053 Carlton VIC

Tel: switchboard (61) (3) 93451800

Fax: (61) (3) 93482513

E-mail: redcross@nat.redcross.org.au

www.redcross.org.au

Canada

170 Metcalfe Street, Suite 300 Ottawa, Ontario K2P 2P2

Tel: (1) (613) 7401900

Fax: (1) (613) 7401911

Telex: CANCROSS 05-33784

E-mail: cancross@redcross.ca

www.redcross.ca

Hong Kong

3 Harcourt Road, Wanchai, Hong Kong

Tel: (852) 28020021

E-mail: hcs@redcross.org.hk

www.redcross.org.hk

India

Red Cross, Building 1, Red Cross Road, 110001 New Delhi

Tel: (91) (112) 371 64 24

Fax: (91) (112) 371 74 54

E-mail: indcross@vsnl.com

www.indianredcross.org

Malaysia
JKR 32, Jalan Nipah, Off Jalan Ampang, 55000 Kuala Lumpur
Tel: (60) (3) 42578122/42578236/42578348/
42578159/42578227
Fax: (60) (3) 42533191
E-mail: mrcs@po.jaring.my
www.redcrescent.org.my

New Zealand
69 Molesworth Street, Thorndon, Wellington
Tel: (64) (4) 4723750
Fax: (64) (4) 4730315
E-mail: national@redcross.org.nz
www.redcross.org.nz

Singapore
Red Cross House, 15 Penang Lane, 238486 Singapore
Tel: (65) 6 3360269
Fax: (65) 6 3374360
E-mail: redcross@starhub.net.sg
www.redcross.org.sg

South Africa
1st Floor, Helen Bowden Building, Beach Road, Granger Bay,
8002 Cape Town
Tel: (27) (21) 4186640
Fax: (27) (21) 4186644
E-mail: sarcs@redcross.org.za
www.redcross.org.za

Taiwan and China
No: 8 Beixingiao Santiao, Dongcheng, East City District,
100007 Beijing
Tel: (86) (10) 8402 5890
Fax: (86) (10) 6406 0566/9928
E-mail: rcsc@chineseredcross.org.cn
www.redcross.org.cn

index

A
ABC checks
and drowning 58
and electrocution 57
and road traffic accidents 54, 55
see also DRABC procedure
abdominal thrusts 34, 35, 36, 37, 68
airway
checking 4
and road traffic accidents 55
choking and blocked airway 32, 35
'finger sweep' 16
opening 14–16
ensuring it stays open 18
alarms, and burning buildings 51
alcohol
and drowning 57
and persons in shock 45
ambulances *see* emergency services
Andrea's story 63–6
anxiety 8–9
approaching emergency situations 1–11
anxiety 8–9
calling the emergency services 3, 7–8, 50
common scenarios 2–3
DRABC procedure 3–5
ensuring safety 6, 10
managing the situation 6–7
self-testers 11
summary 8
aspirin, and heart attacks 59
B
back slaps for choking 33–4, 36, 37, 67, 68
bandaging, around embedded objects 43
bleeding *see* severe bleeding
blood circulation *see* circulation
blood loss
effects of 39
and shock 43–5
and type of wound 39–40, 70
breathing 5
checking for 16–17
and road traffic accidents 55
choking and difficulty in 32, 67, 68
and clinical shock 43
see also rescue breathing
British Red Cross vii, 79–81
first-aid kits 71–4, 75–7
burning buildings 51–2
escaping from 51–2
smoke-filled 52, 53
burning cars 52
burns, treatment of 52
bystanders
and burning cars 52
calling the emergency services 64, 65
and CPR 27
ensuring safety of 10
help from 6

C
car crashes *see* road traffic accidents
Cardio Pulmonary Resuscitation *see* CPR (Cardio Pulmonary Resuscitation)
cars, fires in 52
chest compressions 23, 24–7
  and choking 35, 37
  and CPR 27, 28
  hand position 25, 26
  and the heart 27
  key skills 25
choking 32–38
  abdominal thrusts 34, 35, 36, 37, 68
  back slaps 33–4, 36, 37, 67, 68
  checking the mouth 33, 34, 37
  and chest compressions 35
  and difficulty in breathing 32, 67, 68
  encouraging coughing 32–3, 36, 37
  gagging 32
  Graham's story 66–8
  key skills 36
  self-testers 38
  summary 36–7
  treating 32–5
  and unconsciousness 35, 36
circuit breakers 56
circulation 5
  checking for signs of 23–4, 29
  and chest compressions 27
clinical shock *see* shock
clothes on fire 53–4
cold water, and burns 52
common emergency situations 50–61
  drowning 1, 3, 57–8
  electrical injuries 1, 56–7
  fires 1, 51–4
  heart attacks 58–60
  road traffic accidents 1, 54–6
  self-testers 60–1
coughing, and choking 32–3, 36, 37, 67
CPR (Cardio Pulmonary Resuscitation) 27, 28, 29, 30, 35
  Andrea's story 63–4, 65
cuts, blood loss from 40
D
danger
  assessing 3
  unacceptable risks 3, 50
  see also infection risks
defibrilators 27
diabetes 12
disposable gloves 46
DIY, and electrical injuries 56
DRABC procedure 3–5, 9
  and unconsciousness 12
dressings, applying to wounds 40, 41
drowning 1, 3, 57–8
drugs, and drowning 57
E
electrical injuries 1, 56–7
elevation
  of legs in cases of clinical shock 44, 45
  of wounds 40, 41, 47, 48, 69
emergency services
  and bystanders 64, 65
  calling 3, 7–8, 50

and chest compressions 27
and choking adults 36
and clinical shock 44
and drowning 58
and fires 51, 52
and heart attacks 58–9
and road traffic accidents 54
and severe bleeding 42, 44, 48, 69
and unconscious persons 21, 28, 29
emergency situations *see* common emergency situations
evacuation, of burning buildings 51

F

face shields 23, 63–4, 66
'finger sweep' 16
fire service, and road traffic accidents 54
fire wardens 51
fires 1, 51–4
burning buildings 51–2, 53
clothes on fire 53–4
key skills 52, 54
raising the alarm 51
treating burns 52
first-aid kits 71–4, 75–7
fish bones, choking on 66–8

G

gardening accidents 56
glass, wounds caused by 42–3
gloves, disposable 46
Graham's story 66–8

H

handkerchiefs, and smoke inhalation 53
head injuries 12
the heart
and chest compressions 27
see also elevation
heart attacks 58–60
and aspirin 59
key skills 60
hedge trimmers 56
Heimlich manoeuvre *see* abdominal thrusts
helmets, removing from motorcyclists 55
hospital admissions
choking 68
severe bleeding 69
hypothermia 58

I

infection risks
and rescue breathing 23, 66
and severe bleeding 40, 46
internal bleeding 40
International Red Cross vii, 79, 80
contact details 84–6
International Red Cross and Red Crescent Movement vii, 79–80, 84–6

K

'kiss of life' *see* rescue breathing
knife-related injuries 42–3, 69–70

L

leg wounds 40

M

motorcyclists, and road traffic accidents 55
mouth to mouth ventilation *see* rescue breathing
mowers 56

N
National Red Cross and National Red Crescent Societies 81
O
oxygen 4, 5
P
police, and road traffic accidents 54
pressure, applying to wounds 40, 41, 42, 46, 47, 48
pulse
  checking 24
  and clinical shock 43
R
Raj's story 69–70
recovery position 16, 18–20, 28, 29
rescue breathing 21–3, 29
  and chest compressions 25, 26
  and choking 35
  and face shields 23, 63–4, 66
  giving rescue breaths 22
  key movement in the casualty 22
  key skills 23
  number of attempts at 22
  and risk of infection 23
  unpleasantness of 65
response, checking for 3, 13, 29
resuscitation
  and choking adults 36
  see also CPR (Cardio Pulmonary Resuscitation)
risks
  unacceptable 3, 50
  see also infection risks
road traffic accidents 1, 54–6
  ABC check 54, 55
  calling the emergency services 54
  dangers 3, 6
  key skills 56
  motorcyclists 55
  securing the scene 54
  and unconscious casualties 55
S
safety, and fires 51–2
scalp, blood loss from 40
severe bleeding 39–49
  applying direct pressure to the wound 40, 41, 42, 46, 47, 48, 70
  calling the emergency services 42, 44, 48, 69
  effects of blood loss 39
  elevating the wound 40, 41, 47, 48, 69
  leg wounds 40
  objects embedded in the wound 42–3
  Raj's story 69–70
  and risk of infection 40, 46
  securing pad or dressing 40, 41
  self-testers 49
  and shock 40, 43–5, 48
  summary 47–8
  and tourniquets 42
  and type of wound 39–40
shock
  drinking tea or alcohol 45
  recognizing clinical shock 43–4
  and severe bleeding 40, 43–5
  treating 44–5
    key skills 46
smoke inhalation 52, 53
Stop, Drop, Wrap and Roll

technique 53, 54
stroke 12
surgery, removing embedded objects 43

T

tea, and persons in shock 45
tourniquets 42

U

unacceptable risks 50
unconscious person 12–31
  Andrea's story 63–6
  calling for help 13
  causes of 12
  checking for breathing 16–17
  checking responsiveness 3, 13, 29
  checking for signs of circulation 23–4
  chest compressions 23, 24–7
  choking 35, 36
  and clinical shock 44
  determining 3–4
  key skills 17
  opening the airway 14–16
  placing in the recovery position 16, 18–20, 28, 29
  rescue breathing 21–3
  and road traffic accidents 55
  self–testers 30–1
  summary 28–9

V

varicose veins, and blood loss 40
vomiting
  and clinical shock 44
  and drowning 58
  and rescue breathing 63–4, 66

W

waterproof dressings 46
work, fires at 51–2
wounds
  applying pressure to 40, 41, 42, 46, 47, 48, 70
  and blood loss 39–40, 70
  and dangers of infection 46
  elevating 40, 41, 47, 69
  knife-related injuries 42–3, 69–70
  objects embedded in 42–3
  see also severe bleeding
wrist wounds 69–70